Ten Poses of Yoga

Memory Book

CAMREON DYER

iUniverse LLC
Bloomington

TEN POSES OF YOGA
MEMORY BOOK

iUniverse books may be ordered through booksellers or by contacting:

iUniverse LLC
1663 Liberty Drive
Bloomington, IN 47403
www.iuniverse.com
1-800-Authors (1-800-288-4677)

ISBN: 978-1-4917-2437-8 (sc)
ISBN: 978-1-4917-2438-5 (e)

Library of Congress Control Number: 2014902599

Printed in the United States of America.

iUniverse rev. date: 02/11/2014

Cover photo photographed and edited by
Andrew Miller Photography

All other photos photographed
by Shaylynn Johnson
&
Edited by Andre Santana

Contents

Author's Note

- This book was created to help inspire you, possibly turning you into a future yogi/yogini. Yogi and yogini are related terms to describe a person who is a practioner of Yogic direction. A person who lives with no limits and knows that no matter what god has the last say. Far from being a gender tag to all things this book is for any race, any shape, all sizes, and all people. It is purposely written so that everyone can understand each pose step by step. You could think of it as "yoga for dummies," but we all know that anyone who is a yogini is far from a dummy! The world is full of excuses for why you should or should not practice yoga. The definition of Yoga means union, communion; meaning to join or yoke as one. Yoga has been around for years, but the next generation yoginis have taken it to another level, making it especially popular in urban society. Yoga is a very motivational experience within itself, inspiring people to live healthier life styles. People go through so much in their lives that yoga is sometimes used as an outlet to get over difficulties and challenges. Use this memory book to inspire you to practice different poses and insert photos to remember. Please feel free to post your pictures on our Instagram page @CambellaYoga to comment on and share your journey. Yoga is a FULL experience—faith, unity, loyalty, longevity. Let the poses begin.

Acknowledgments

We all have dreams. I am aware that the patience of success is overcoming stereotypes and challenging one's mental state of mind and body. In our homes today, as always, life is centered on the human body. To achieve anything in life requires faith, and I am willing to except criticism in order to excel. I wouldn't have been able to do this if it wasn't for you; I dedicate this book to all yoginis and the 608 asanas (yoga poses). To my family and friends, I want express my gratitude to you all for giving me the ability to create a masterpiece of my own.

Once more, I appreciate my sisters, Shaylynn Johnson and Chasity Workman, for believing in me and being there for me along this journey. I hope you enjoy the outstanding quotes and my treasured poses.

Inspiration

One day I was scrolling through Instagram, and I saw a pose that caught my eye and had me in awe. I said to myself, *Wow, I have to try this*. I hurried home after work to attempt the pose because I knew that I could do it. I jumped straight into the pose without any stretching. I had not done yoga in years, but without practice I jumped right into it on my first attempt. The excitement of actually doing it gave me an instant rush that I enjoyed. A week later, I attempted it again, and I couldn't do it. I couldn't figure out how I was able to do it one week and not the next. Yoga intrigued me so much that I decided to study it.

People think that just because they can do a pose that they are practicing yoga, but that's not the case. The greatest thing about being a yogini is that when you start to practice, you get a high that has you so FULL that the sensation gives you a rush of pure energy, mentally stimulating thoughts that you are capable of doing anything. Yoga uses a holistic approach that is both psychological and physical. Breaking up each step involves comprehending the pose as a whole. I've learned that the mind is more powerful than anything physical in life.

People on Instagram and Facebook, actually practicing and doing yoga, inspired me to create this book. I have a degree in psychology, and through research I was able to determine that yoga therapy has a lot to do with helping cure mental illness and also decreases stress. Yoga is a very beautiful form of art performed and created by the human body. This is not a simple task but is accomplished because of one's strong mind. Increasing self-awareness means focusing on present, reducing negative emotions, controlling breathing, and having a calm mind that requires concentration and balance; focus less on your day and more on the moment.

My mother is forty-six years old has experienced breast cancer and a brain turmor. At first she was hesitant about practicing yoga because of everything she has been through. The thing is in life we go through life, and no matter what your problems are you have to still continue to live! Yoga means one with self and God. I was able to inspire my mother to practice yoga not only because of her health but also because the practice of merging yoga with faith and god; which is done through mental, spiritual and physical practices.

Start off slowly with stretches and small workouts. Also do lots of breathing techniques and regular stretches. Most of these poses aren't as difficult as they seem, and the focus is more on balance and concentration. Learn to get rid of nervous tension. The key is to get your mind to work for you and not against you.

The second step is to get rid of your expectations for a pose. No pose is perfect; if you learn not to expect anything, then you have mastered perfection. However, if you haven't done any workouts in years, don't think that these poses will be easy on a first attempt. Yoga helps you with many different things, such as digestion, strength, flexibility, relationships, weight loss, and breathing. Yoga is process that needs to be practiced at least once a day.

Daily Exercises

- The low-impact stretches you do before any workout will help you get into more of the Ashtanga yoga poses. Ashtanga is a system of exercises practiced as part of this discipline to promote control of the body and mind. Most simple stretches need to be done at least once a day. For example, you should do these stretches daily: shoulder rolls, torso twist, torso circles, touching your toes from right to left, stretching yours arms from right to left. This is important if you want to become more flexible.

Introduction

- Start off with some warm-ups.
- Do some low-impact stretches.
- Read your quote before and after your practice/poses.
- Once you get comfortable in the pose, take a photo and insert it in the slot.
- Fill up your memory book. If you're comfortable, post it on our website.

Sitting Pose of the Sage Durva

Sometimes yoga can distract you from or decrease life's anxieties. Different stretching techniques can help avoid distress. Yoga inspires you to go beyond your limitations mentally, physically, and emotionally, allowing the mind to be free. Your physical and mental health will benefit.

- Lie flat on your back.
- Have your knees up.
- Take your right leg and put it behind your head.
- Take your left arm and hold your right foot.
- Take your right arm and place it underneath, crossing your right leg, until your elbow is touching the floor.

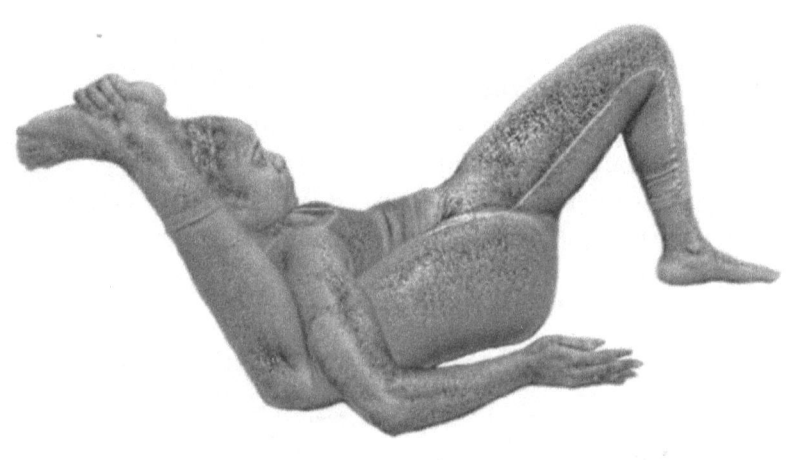

Sleeping Hero

*Release negative thoughts of what you can't do, and
move beyond the fear of what you can.*

- Sit on your knees.
- Lie straight back, head on the floor.
- Push your shoulders up with your head on the crown.
- Reach your arms straight out, side by side on your thighs.

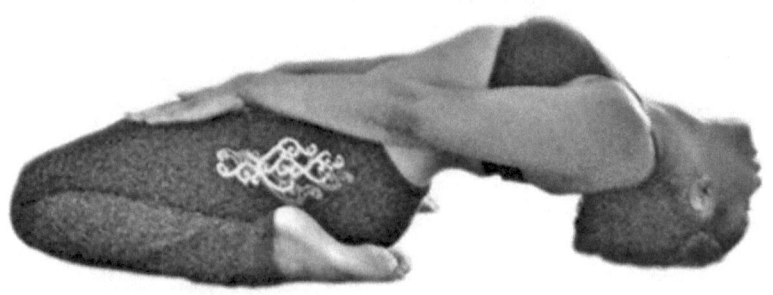

Hands-Free Headstand Pose

Breathe. Know that nothing can stop you but you.

*This is an advanced pose.

- Place your book in front of you.
- Slowly go into a headstand.
- Hold your legs straight upward.
- Bending the left leg will help with balance.
- Slowly grab your book and try to read two pages.

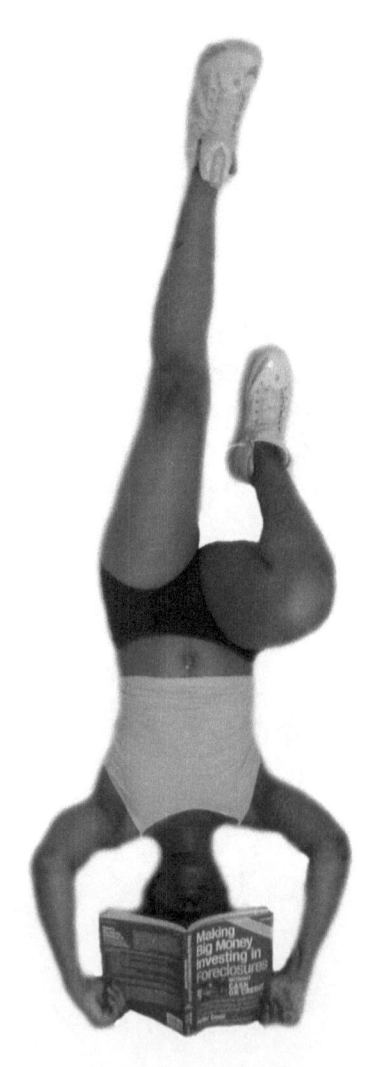

One Leg Scorpion Pose

It's time to do something new; don't put limits on what you can do physically by never putting in your mind that you could do it mentally.

- Start by practicing on or between a wall or doorway.
- Make sure your hands are at least 2 feet away.
- Place your hands on the floor.
- Take your right leg and place it on the wall. Walk both legs upward.
- Stretch your right leg backward.

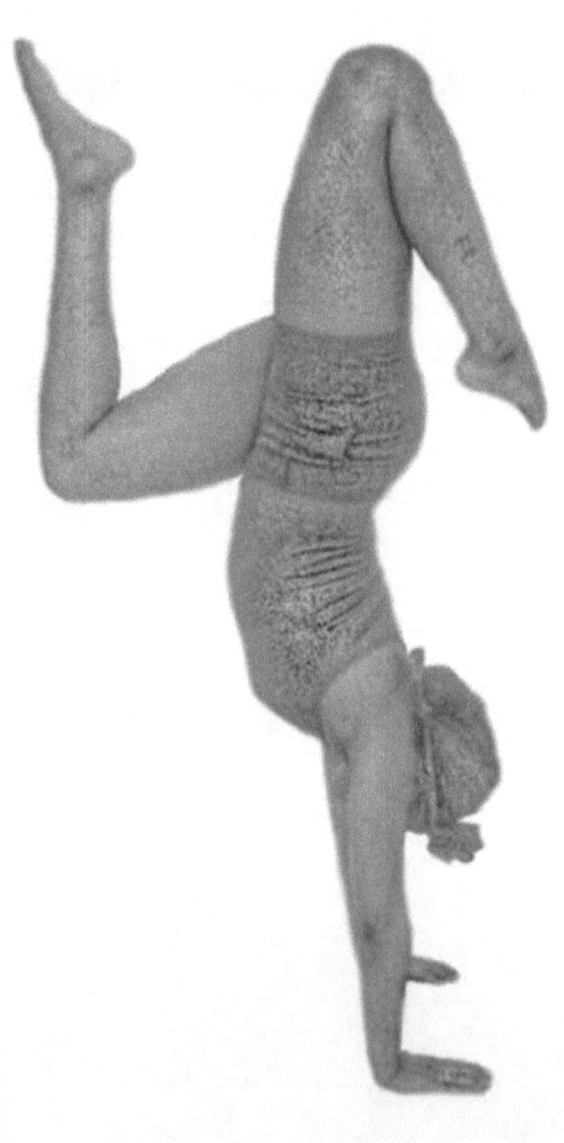

One Leg Inverted Staff Pose

We all have to start somewhere; just because you can't do it today doesn't mean you won't be able to do it tomorrow.

- Lie flat on your back.
- Put your arms in the air and bend them.
- Tuck your arms toward your back.
- Push up on the tips of your toes.
- Push your chest upward.
- Take your right leg off the ground and point your toes.

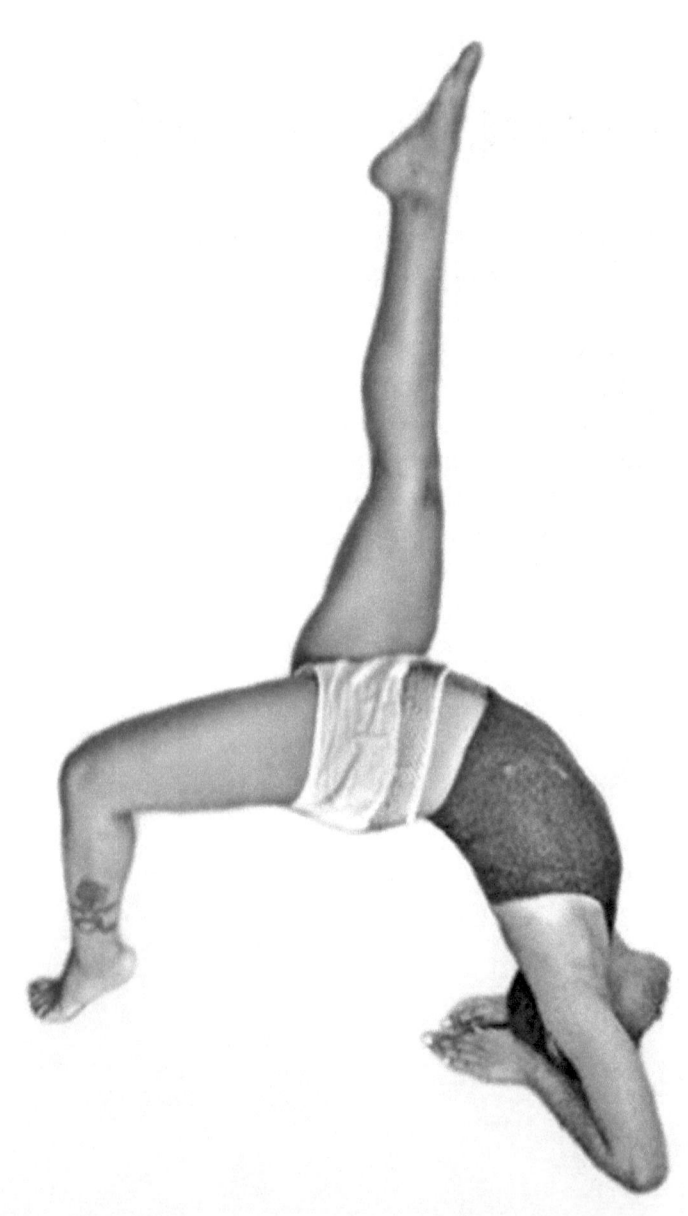

Downward-Facing Tree Pose

All things are possible, no matter how slow you go, as long as every day you improve as a person (mentally and physically).

- Place both feet together.
- Bend over and touch your feet.
- Take your right leg, grab your foot, and extend it out.
- Make sure your arm and leg are straight.
- Hold the pose.

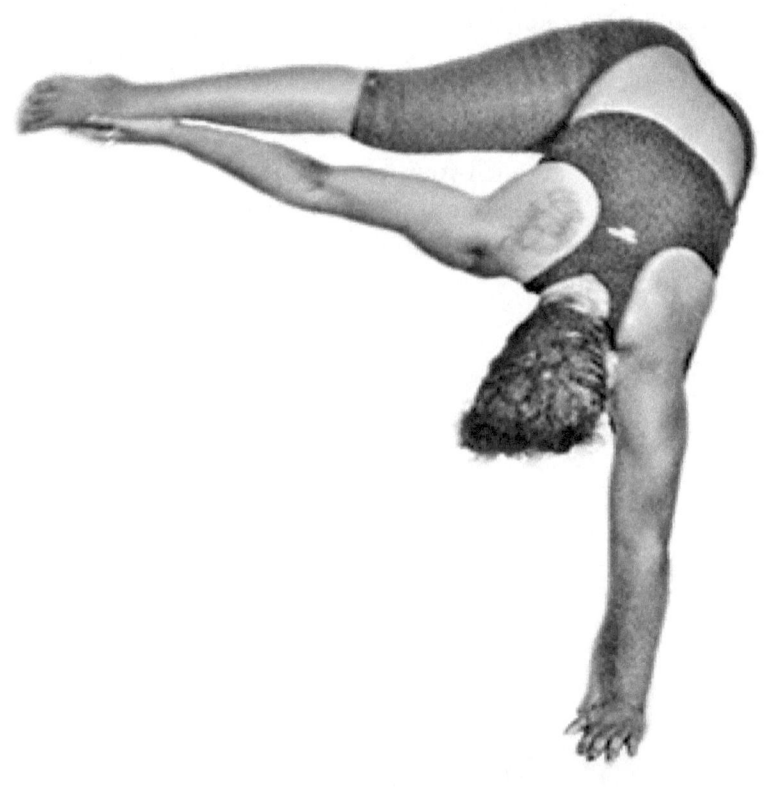

Pose 8

Focus. Realize that your mind is a muscle. It is not weak. The more you exercise it, the stronger it becomes. You can overcome all obstacles.

*This is an advanced pose.

- Lie flat on your back.
- Lift your torso into an upward position.
- Bend your right leg and point your toes.
- Grab your left foot with your left arm.
- Breathe.

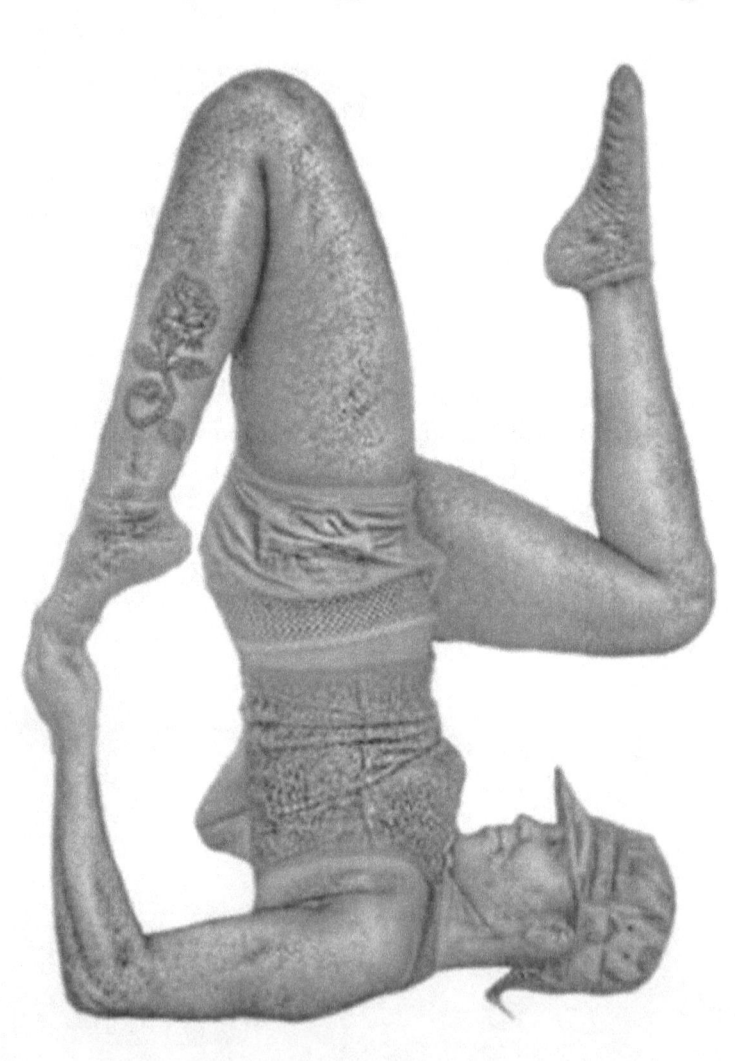

Dancer's Pose

Explore. Laziness does not exist. Place yourself in the mental state that you are capable of moving mountains.

*This can be done on either leg, whichever one is more comfortable.

- Balance on one leg, bend the other knee, and grasp your foot.
- Bring the foot and opposite arm upward.
- Lean forward and stretch your other arm straight out.

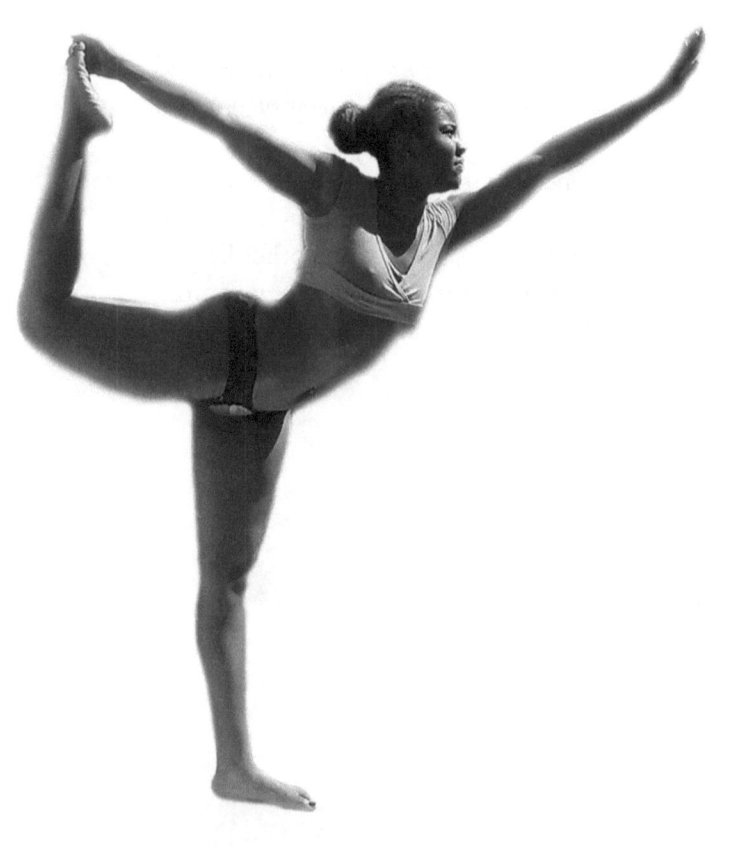

Spread-Out-Leg Intense Stretch Pose

Relax. No one is perfect, no sport is perfect, no pose is perfect, and yoga isn't perfect. Perfection is the opportunity presented in one's self.

- Stand up straight.
- Take both arms and reach behind you.
- Take both hands and put them together.
- Spread both legs.
- Bend over slowly; keep going until your head is touching the floor.

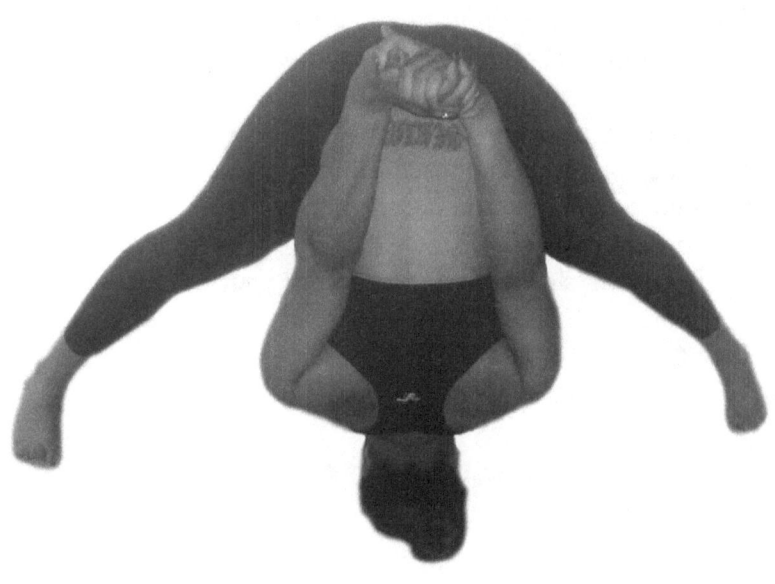

Upward Plough Head Pose

Breathe, relax, focus, explore. Open your mind. There's so much more to life than just the core. Look deeper inside yourself. Take some time to get to know you.

- Stand up straight.
- Take both arms and reach behind you.
- Take both hands and put them together.
- Spread both legs.
- Bend over slowly; keep going until your head is touching the floor.
- Slowly walk both feet together.
- Push both arms up in the air.

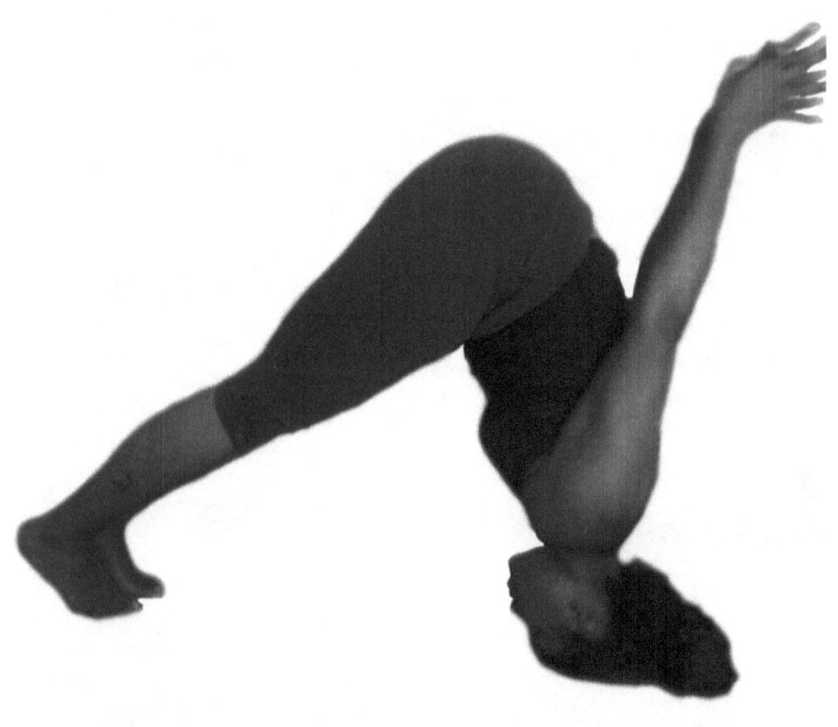

Yoga food for thought: Mind and body, inspiration, education, and spirit.

I thank all those who generously gave their words of encouragement and inspirational feedback. Without your help this book would have never been possible.

To all my family and friends I just want to say thank you for all your support. A lot of you have been asking me questions about if yoga also helps enhance my personal relationship, well the answer is yes. I want to introduce you all to my new book *Yoga is Art: Imagination can save Sex.* Is a book on How to add stimulation and creativity to your relationship. Becoming more flexible increases the chances of your partner staying interested; making your sex life that much more exciting. If you are open minded and receptive to new things then you are more likely to keep your partners attention and that is the key. Open your minds to transform your relationships into an incredibly intimate erotic event.

Scorpion Partner Pose

People are visual, In relationships naughty and nice have no definition in the bedroom

- Start off practicing on a wall, chair or your partner
- Practice bending and stretching your back
- Hands separated flat on the floor forearm stand
- Make sure at least a foot from the wall
- Kick your legs up towards the wall
- Walking both feet down towards your head
- Lift your head up

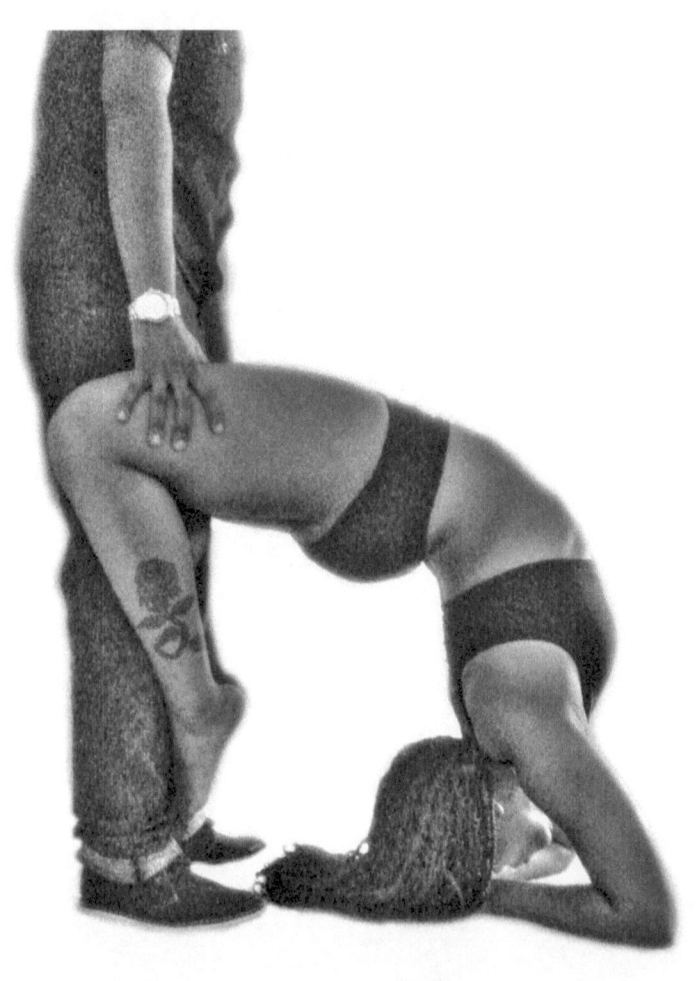

Coming Soon

www.ingramcontent.com/pod-product-compliance
Lightning Source LLC
Chambersburg PA
CBHW030529290526
45786CB00004B/1661